LIVING LONGER

A PROVEN PLAN FOR A LONG, HEALTHY, AND ACTIVE LIFE

Edited by Wayne Purdin
Front cover design by VirtualElf LLC
Back cover and spine design by 100covers

CONTENTS

TAKING CONTROL

Do you think that longevity is just a matter of luck? Do you feel that staying healthy for life is not realistic? Do you believe that it is normal to become weak and sick as you grow older?

What if I told you it's never too late to take control of your health and wellness regardless of whether you are in your thirties, forties, fifties, sixties or seventies?

What if I told you that genetics is just a small component of longevity? That you have significant control over how long you live and how active your life can be?

What if I showed you that it's possible to take control of your chronic conditions and enhance your sense of well-being without making unpleasant lifestyle changes?

What if I convinced you that slowing down with age is not natural for the human body? That our bodies are designed to be healthy, strong and vital for long as we live?

Are you willing to spend a few hours reading this book? Are you ready to change your life?

Chapter 1:
LONGEVITY IS THE NEW NORMAL

---

*A long and healthy life is not a miracle.
It just requires a plan.*

It is official. Humans are living longer, in larger numbers than ever before!

The Pew Research Center published a paper in 2015 which showed that the number of Centenarians in the world has increased four-fold from the year 2000 to the year 2015. That paper also stated that there will be eight times more Centenarians by the year 2050. Obviously, humanity is going in the right direction!

What are the reasons for this incredible accomplishment? We know that the increase in lifespan is not a smooth curve, but it came in spurts with Humanity conquering multiple thresholds. Our key to living longer is to understand what these thresholds are, how we overcame these thresholds, and incorporate that understanding into our lives.

Without further ado, here are the thresholds:

THRESHOLD ONE

The distinction of being the first threshold belongs to infectious diseases. We all know from history that infections like bubonic plague, cholera, typhoid used to wipe out entire villages and towns. In 1918, the Spanish flu killed more than twenty million people. Humanity paid a heavy price due to infections, and the average lifespan back then was in the high twenties.

Over time, we invented vaccinations and antibiotics. While new infections like SARS and COVID-19 continue to ravage us, we have figured out how to collaborate globally and bring these killer infections under quick control every time we have a new one popping up. The immunization strategies we have created have pushed human lifespan by a good thirty years from the high twenties to high fifties.

However, we can only take advantage of these incredible accomplishments by being proactive with immunizations for ourselves and our families. Anytime a new contagion or infection breaks out, we also need to be proactive about following safe distancing guidelines, lockdowns and other temporary measures to stay safe while giving time for researchers to discover new vaccines or other cures to combat that new threat.

It is very easy to stay up to date with your immunizations and prevention strategies. Among the many things you can do to enhance your lifespan, this is the lowest hanging fruit!

THRESHOLD TWO

Since we have removed infections as the biggest killer of humanity, other killers have taken up that place. According to a recent list published by the Center of Disease Control, the leading causes of death today are Heart Disease, Cancer, Accidents, Chronic respiratory diseases, Stroke, Alzheimer's disease and Diabetes. These leading causes are the second threshold we need to talk about.

There is still no cure for many of these problems. However, rapid advances in healthcare and wellness strategies have provided us excellent ways to manage these problems and reduce their impacts on our lifespan. These advances have increased humanity's average lifespan from high fifties to high seventies.

So, managing this second threshold effectively can increase your lifespan by a good twenty plus years. This is however a little more difficult than managing the first threshold. You need access to good healthcare which can be expensive. It takes tedious work, a good partnership with your doctors and other professionals in order to detect problems early on, and come up with effective strategies to manage them.

THRESHOLD THREE

This threshold belongs to lifestyle. Effective management of weight, nutrition, physical activity and stress has been proven to provide substantial gains in lifespan.

Luckily, there is enormous research being done in this area. The Blue Zones Project is one such example where lifestyles of some of the longest-lived people on earth have been studied. In general, there is incredible information, knowhow and help available for us to make smarter lifestyle choices and expand our lifespans by a good twenty plus years!

Unfortunately, most lifestyle changes require will power, discipline and determination to sustain. This is where most people fail. Some folks make new lifestyle resolutions every year only to give them up after a few months. The secret to making lifestyle improvements sustainable is to make them a natural part of your life, in a way that they do not require special efforts to maintain.

THRESHOLD FOUR

This last threshold is life itself. Basically, keeping up with the steps to combat the first three thresholds described above requires resources and tedious efforts. Most people do not have a plan that is comprehensive and flexible enough to keep up with these, because life gets in the way.

The secret to making your longevity plan sustainable over the long term is to make it automated, flexible, practical, easy and addictive. Managing this last threshold well gives you the best chance to overcome any last impediments to living beyond a hundred years and making those years memorable!

A FOUR-STEP PLAN
FOR LONGEVITY

The four thresholds described above gives us a comprehensive idea of why more and more people are succeeding in living longer and healthier lives. Research shows that people who are reaching the magic goal of being Centenarians are indeed managing these four thresholds well, whether it is because their environments give them a natural path to do so, or they developed that path on their own.

The four thresholds also explain why more than ninety-nine percent of the world population is failing to reach that goal of living beyond a hundred years. Basically, most people do not have a comprehensive plan that addresses all four thresholds effectively, which is why they fail in one stage or another.

This is the reason why I wrote this book. I have worked for many years in the healthcare industry, and I have learnt that living a long and healthy life is possible, but it requires a solid plan.

Basically, your longevity plan boils down to a four-step plan described below that effectively manages the four thresholds described above. This four-step plan brings together a blend of latest best practices, medical advancements, lifestyle improvement techniques and technological advancements into one simple solution. It packs everything we know about longevity into one package that is easy to follow and sustainable over time.

Here is the four-step plan:

The Four Steps	Description of each step
Step 1: **FOUNDATION**	This step is about laying basic foundational blocks like selecting the right health coverage, optimizing your access to primary care

Step 2: **INTERVENTION**	This step is about effective risk management. It is about
Step 3: **PREVENTION**	This step is about making smart life choices that keep you younger, make you stronger and help you live longer.
Step 4: **AUTOMATION**	The three steps above make up your longevity plan, and have a lot of details

These four steps above are very flexible. They cover a wide range of scenarios as follows:

1. They are suitable for people with a wide variety of lifestyles and income levels.
2. They work for all age groups and ethnicities.
3. They work for people who live in different geographies and climates.
4. This framework adapts and stays current as our knowledge improves in all the four threshold areas described above.
5. Once you have this four-step plan up and running, you will set yourself up for a significantly higher quality of life, with better control over your health, wellness and longevity.

In the following chapters, I describe each of these four steps in detail, provide you checklists and other tools that make them easy to implement and sustain.

Let us move on to Step 1. Happy reading!

FOUNDATION

Longevity favors people who are best prepared. This step is about laying the foundation blocks for supporting a long, healthy and happy lifestyle.

Chapter 2
AFFORDABLE ACCESS TO CARE

For leading a long and healthy life, some medical interventions may be necessary along the way. In today's world, medical intervention can be expensive. Having access to affordable care is an important foundational block for your longevity plan.

I remember the joyful time when my first kid was born. I also vividly remember what followed next, which was an unending series of medical bills end expenses. I met with my benefits coordinator in my office and discussed why I was paying so much money out of pocket.

I discovered that when I got married, I had simply added my spouse to the health insurance plan I had when I was single, without reviewing the coverages or selecting a different plan to adjust for changed conditions. Instead, If I had sat down and reviewed my coverages, selected a plan more suitable for a young family, I would have saved a substantial amount of money during the times that followed!

My woes were not caused because I lacked access to the right medical plans. It was caused because I was careless and did not do my part in making the right selections at the right time.

Your needs for medical coverage can change over time. It is necessary to review your needs periodically and adjust your coverage so that you always take best advantage of the benefits available to you. This is how you keep your costs low and optimize your coverage.

Making sure you have the right kind of coverages is a multi-step process. Let us go through this one step at a time. When it comes to Healthcare, every country does it differently. The steps below are mostly geared for United States, but if you live in another country, I am sure you can use this for reference but extrapolate based on how medical coverage works in your country.

STEP 1: ASSESS YOUR CURRENT NEEDS FOR CARE

Your health needs change all the time. It is necessary to understand your ongoing needs especially when there are life changes, and adjust your coverages. The nature of the coverage you need depends on your answers to the following questions:

- What is your age?
- What is your marital status?
- How many dependents do you have?
- What is your job and income status?
- Is your family in one geographic location, or spread out?
- Are there any recent additions or other changes to your family?
- Do you use tobacco?
- Do you travel a lot?

- Do you travel internationally?
- Do you have pre-existing conditions in your family that need ongoing care?
- Do you need coverage for disabilities or other special needs?

Any time, your answers change for any of these questions, you will need to re-assess your healthcare needs.

STEP 2: REVIEW YOUR COVERAGE OPTIONS

Now that you have a basic idea of your needs, it is time to review the coverage options that are available to you. Sometimes, based on your needs, you may be able to access more than one option.

For example, you and your spouse may have separate health coverages. You may have additional coverage because of veteran benefits, Medicare, etc. It is necessary to take a holistic look at all the available options, examples of which are below:

- **Employer provided health insurance:** Most employers offer insurance options for employees where the employer pays a part of the subscription cost and the employee pays the remaining part. Generally, you will have several choices depending on your situation.

- **Short-term health insurance:** This is a type of health plan that can provide you with temporary medical coverage when you are between health plans or outside enrollment periods, and need some coverage in case of an emergency.

- **Medicare:** Medicare is a federal health insurance program for people age 65 or older, younger people with disabilities and people with permanent kidney failure requiring dialysis or transplant. It has two parts, Part A (Hospital Insurance) and Part B (Medicare Insurance).

- **Medicaid:** This is a healthcare program that assists low-income families or individuals in paying for doctor visits, hospital stays, long-term medical, custodial care costs and more. Medicaid is a joint program, funded primarily by the federal government and run at the state level, where coverage may vary.

- **On-exchange private health insurance:** On-exchange means the plans that are available through government-created marketplaces, like the federal marketplace (Healthcare.gov) or a state marketplace, like MNsure in Minnesota. Shopping on-exchange is a great option if you qualify for some subsidies that can be applied towards your coverages.

- **Off-exchange private health insurance:** This term refers to insurance plans that are not offered on public marketplaces but you can purchase them through private insurance carriers or licensed brokers. This is a good option if you do not have other kinds of coverages listed above.

Depending on your situation, find out which of the options above you are eligible for.

STEP 3: PICK THE RIGHT INSURANCE TYPE

You have just reviewed your coverage options. Within each of these options, there are usually several insurance types available. Here are some of the types possibly available to you:

- **HMO (Health Maintenance Organization):** This kind of coverage is meant to provide you a wider range of preventative healthcare services within a network of providers at a lower cost. However, it is restrictive, and you can see specialists only with referral from your primary care physician. This kind of coverage is great if you are generally healthy and need basic, preventative services including easy access to primary care.

- **PPO (Preferred Provider Organization):** PPO is a more premium form of coverage. These plans allow you to visit whichever specialist you need within a network of physicians, without first requiring a referral from a primary care physician. This is a better coverage if you or your family have health conditions that require more specialized care. If you need to go outside of your preferred network, coverage is still available but you may need to bear a larger burden of costs.

- **EPO (Exclusive Provider Organization):** EPO is an exclusive network like a hospital chain. As a member of an EPO, you can use the doctors and hospitals within the EPO network, but cannot go outside the network for care. There are no out-of-network benefits.

- **POS (Point of Service):** This is a hybrid of HMO and PPO plans. Like an HMO, participants designate an in-network physician to be their primary care provider. But like a PPO, patients may go outside of the provider network for health care services.

Based on the needs for you and your dependents, select the type that makes most sense for now. Keep in mind your needs can change over time.

STEP 4: BE AWARE OF YOUR PREFERRED PROVIDER NETWORK

Once you have selected your option and type, your insurance carrier will make available to you a 'preferred providers' list that gives you access to a wide variety of specialties. Please refer to this list before you go see a doctor. Seeing physicians outside of this preferred list will increase your costs significantly.

Some insurances have a wide geographic coverage. Others are more local or regional. If you have a regional coverage, find out from your provider what your options are if you travel out of that geographic range. If you travel internationally, find out from your insurance provider what your coverage options are. In most cases, you may need to buy a supplemental insurance or pay out of pocket for international coverage.

STEP 5: UNDERSTAND YOUR OUT-OF-POCKET EXPENSES

Depending on the insurance option and type you select, your out of out-of-pocket expenses may vary widely.

Here are the most common out-of-pocket expenses:

- **Premium:** This is the monthly payment you make to buy the medical coverage you are interested in.

- **Deductible:** The deductible is the amount of money you will pay out of pocket before the insurance coverage kicks in and starts paying for covered services.

- **Copayment:** A copayment is a fixed amount you pay every time you receive service. If your copay is $20, then you pay $20 every time you see a doctor after the deductible is satisfied. The insurance covers the rest of the cost for that service.

- **Coinsurance:** This is the percentage of the cost of a covered service you pay (20%, for example) after you've paid your deductible. Let's say your health insurance plan's allowed amount for an office visit is $100 and your coinsurance is 20%. If you've paid your deductible: You pay 20% of $100, or $20.

- **Maximum out-of-pocket amount:** This is the most you need to pay for covered services in a plan year. After you spend this amount on deductibles, copayments, and coinsurance, your health plan pays 100% of the costs of covered benefits. Your monthly premium is not included in this consideration.

Before you consult a medical professional or undergo a procedure or a diagnostic test, you have a right to know what your out of pocket expenses are going to be. Make sure you understand your expenses to avoid unpleasant financial surprises!

STEP 6: UNDERSTAND YOUR SUPPLEMENTAL COVERAGE NEEDS

Sometimes, your primary insurance may not cover some of your needs effectively, Case in point, seniors that have MEDICARE may frequently seek additional coverages if they have some pre-exiting conditions. Here are some examples of supplemental plans. Evaluate of you need any such plans:

- Dental insurance for adults
- Critical Illness Insurance
- Vision Insurance Plans
- Disability Insurance
- Supplemental Travel Insurance for Healthcare coverage
- Long term care insurance
- Short term health insurance coverage
- Medicare or Medicaid Supplemental Plans

STEP 7: UNDERSTAND THE BASIC COVERAGES IN YOUR PLAN

Here are some basic coverages you can expect in most insurance plans:
- Outpatient services
- Emergency services
- Hospitalization for surgery, overnight stays, and other conditions
- Pregnancy, maternity, and newborn care
- Mental health and substance use disorder services
- Prescription drugs
- Rehabilitative and facilitative services and devices
- Laboratory services

- Preventive and wellness services, as well as chronic disease management
- Pediatric services, including dental and vision coverage for children

STEP 8: KNOW THE PREVENTATIVE SCREENINGS AVAILABLE TO YOU

Find out what preventative screenings you can take advantage of, based on your needs. Here is an example list of screenings that insurances typically cover. This is not an exhaustive list. Not everything in this list is relevant all the time, but depending on your age, your condition and family situation, some of these may come in handy during various phases of your life:

- Alcohol misuse screening and counseling
- Blood pressure screening
- Cholesterol screening
- Colorectal cancer screening
- Diet counseling
- Hepatitis B screening
- Hepatitis C screening
- HIV screening
- Statin preventive medication
- Depression screening
- Diabetes (Type 2) screening
- Syphilis screening
- Tobacco use screening and cessation interventions
- Tuberculosis screening
- Immunization vaccines
- Lung cancer screening
- Obesity screening and counseling
- Sexually transmitted infection prevention counseling

STEP 9: UNDERSTAND YOUR WELLNESS OPTIONS

Medical Insurance typically does not pay for lifestyle improvements. For example, health club membership, nutrition consultation, yoga classes, etc.

However, many employers are increasingly realizing that an all-round employee is more than just a healthy employee. They are realizing that employees physical, social, financial and emotional health are all related. Because of this growing awareness, most employers have started offering wellness options that are above and beyond your health insurance coverages. These wellness options can go a long way towards making your life better. Based on your situation, you can take advantage of many wellness programs as below:

- Health club memberships
- Aerobics and weight training consultations
- Diet and nutrition counseling
- Mental and social health services
- Counseling services for developing a sense of connection
- Stress management
- Career planning and financial counseling

This is great for both employers and for us the employees. From employer perspective, taking care of employees helps drive a sense of well-being and higher engagement from them. For employees, it offers a great opportunity to customize the wellness programs to suit your needs for overall improvement end become a more satisfied and happy person.

Find out what your wellness coverages are. Sometimes, this may be the most rewarding part of your compensation package!

CHECKLIST

You have come to the end of Chapter 2. Here is a brief checklist of action items to make sure you have taken the necessary action to reach the goals that you want this book to help you with. It will help you immensely if you complete this checklist before moving on to the next chapter:

MY ACTION ITEMS

Here are my action items based on the recommendations in this chapter:

- I have analyzed my Healthcare needs.
- I have selected the right health plan based on steps described in this chapter.
- I have adjusted the coverages to be optimal for me and my family.
- I have made plans to periodically review my needs and adjust for changes.
- I have taken advantage of the wellness options available to me.

I am ready to move on to the next chapter!

Chapter 3
SETTING UP YOUR TEAM

Longevity is a team sport. There are many highly qualified professionals who are eager to help you live longer, healthier, stronger, happier and more productive lives. Give them a chance, put your health insurance to good use, and make these professionals a part of your life. Having access to a team of qualified professionals is an important foundational block for living a long and successful life.

In the previous chapter, you finished setting up the right medical insurance and wellness coverage options for yourself and family. Now it is time to set up and optimize your access to care. This is your second building block towards building a strong foundation.

Most people see their doctors only when they have a problem. Your approach should be more proactive. You should see your primary care doctors every six to twelve months based on what your insurance allows you to do, regardless of whether you have any problem or not. This helps you create preventative support around you, and address health issues before they become serious problems.

I want to share a situation from when I was a traveling consultant during the first few years of my marriage. My wife and kids were traveling with me. Every two to three years, I had to move my family to a different city. Because we were moving so frequently, our access to healthcare was mostly reactive. We scheduled time with doctors only if one of us felt sick or needed some immunization shots. It was usually a new doctor every time, at some medical institution closest to where we were staying at that time.

Because we were moving frequently, my family never got the opportunity to develop a dedicated network of medical care around us until we settled down. We missed out on having a continuity of care. Once we settled down however, we could create a primary care system around us where the doctors knew us, and could proactively help us stay healthy and avoid diseases.

Setting up a good primary care network around you is an important step towards laying the foundation for proactive health management.

SETTING UP YOUR PRIMARY CARE NETWORK

Start with selecting a primary care medical, dental and vision practitioner from your list of preferred providers. Set up recurring appointments with them. Most insurance plans pay for primary care visits at least once every six months or so. Some lower cost plans pay for the same once every 12 months.

Make sure your choices of practitioners are convenient in terms of easy access, closeness to home or work, etc. Anything that is not convenient will not work in the long run. Also, make sure your primary care providers are transparent, friendly, helpful and willing to answer your questions. Otherwise, pick a different doctor. Remember, you are in charge!

There are several benefits to seeing your primary care providers every six months even if you have no medical conditions requiring you to see them. Here are some benefits:

- Primary care doctors focus on prevention and early detection
- They can run routine checks and refill your medications as needed
- They focus on a holistic approach to health
- You can get referrals to the right specialists quickly when needed
- They provide continuity of care because they get to know you personally

Primary care is simple to set up. It has been statistically proven to provide significant improvements to the health and longevity of your entire family by using a preventative approach to care. This is one of the low hanging fruits that gives you incredible benefits with minimal efforts, because the system is already there and optimized for your use!

SETTING UP YOUR WELLNESS CONNECTIONS

One of the best things you can do for yourself is to set up a network of wellness connections around you. Your well-being is more than just health and physical fitness. Are financial troubles bogging you down? Are you going through stress because of relationships? You will be surprised to find that your employer may be willing to help you in these areas!

Explore and exploit every opportunity you can get for improving your wellness and making life engaging and interesting. There is no point in living long if you cannot live well. Here are some things your employer may be willing to pay for:

- Health club membership
- Aerobics, weights, Pilates or yoga classes
- Nutrition counseling
- Sport club memberships
- Financial planning
- Stress management consultations
- Relationship management consultations

IMMUNIZE YOUR FAMILY

If you are a history buff, you know that whole villages used to be wiped out due to bacterial and viral infections like the flu, typhoid, plague, malaria, etc. Humanity has made huge sacrifices in the past, and thus, we have wonderful vaccines and therapies that can prevent you from ever having to contract these deadly diseases.

It is easy. Your primary care physician will automatically make sure you are up to date with immunizations including the periodic flu vaccine. Just follow your physician's advice.

At the time of writing this book, the world is fighting the deadly COVID-19 virus. While this virus has temporarily destabilized life around the whole world, humanity will eventually create a vaccine and get out of this tragic mess. Therefore, keeping up with immunizations is important. Without immunizations, you will be exposing yourself and your family to unnecessary risks which are easily preventable.

FOLLOW GOVERNMENT ADVISORIES

Since the world is going through COVID-19 infection crisis at the time of writing this book, there is a current government advisory for maintaining social distancing, self-quarantine, using face masks and maintaining hand hygiene. Following these advisories may save you from accidental exposure to the deadly virus, and premature death.

Also, if you travel frequently, it is good to review travel advisories from your Government and be appropriately immunized. Simple measures like these can help avoid unnecessary risks to your health and help you live longer.

INVESTING IN YOURSELF

One of the most important things you can do for yourself is to get a life coach. People who pursue personal growth and push themselves to the limit are usually healthier and happier. You only live once. You get a one-time opportunity to live a fulfilling, productive, and positive life. Embrace it!

Whether your idea of fulfillment comes from playing sports, traveling, writing novels, helping others, you should find that passion and aggressively pursue it. A life coach is professionally trained to help you maximize your full potential and reach your desired results. A life coach can help you with the following:

- Identify, clarify and create a vision for what you want to do to feel fulfilled
- Encourage your self-discovery and growth
- Nurture and evoke strategies and a plan of action based on what fits best with your goals, personality and vision
- Hold you accountable to achieve your goals
- You may find that your employer may pay for something like this as part of a wellness package. Go for it!

CHECKLIST

You have come to the end of Chapter 3. Here is your checklist of action items to make sure you have taken the necessary actions recommended in this chapter:

MY ACTION ITEMS

- I have identified my primary care network.
- I have set up recurring appointments with our primary care providers.
- I have made sure that my family is up to date on all immunizations.
- I commit to keeping up with periodic immunizations like the flu vaccine.
- I have set up my health club membership.
- I commit to following government advisories as needed.
- I have set up my wellness connections based on the options available to me.

I am ready to move on to the next chapter!

INTERVENTION

Proactive management of health, wellness and safety risks can increase the duration and quality of your life

Chapter 4
IDENTIFYING YOUR CHRONIC CONDITIONS

We all have weaknesses that can impact longevity. Probably, some pre-existing health problems like high blood pressure or diabetes. Maybe some harmful addictions like excessive alcohol consumption or drug abuse. Maybe dangerous habits like texting while driving. These weaknesses should be clearly identified so that they can be managed. Effective recognition and management of weaknesses is a key contributor to longevity.

WE ARE ONLY AS STRONG AS OUR WEAKEST LINK

One of my friends, Jason Lee was an avid hiker and body builder. He was an image of fitness, good health and positive attitude. It was always a lot of fun to be around him. And then, at 37, he just passed away one night with no warning, leaving his friends and family bewildered and shattered!

It appeared that he had High Blood Pressure that he refused to manage using regular medications. He had tried dietary approaches and exercise routines to manage this problem without much success.

So, in the end it did not matter how strong he was, how good his diet and exercise routines were, how well-managed his habits were, or how meticulously he managed his stress. The one known weakness he had, his high blood pressure, was enough to bring him down and end his life.

Emily, my son's classmate got a Mercedes Sedan as a Christmas Gift after she turned 17. She was a high school senior at that time with straight A grades and a wonderful extracurricular life, being active in theater and music. Obviously, the proud parents wanted nothing but the best for their daughter!

Two months later, Emily had a head-on collision with another car, and was hospitalized with a broken sternum and internal bleeding. Luckily she survived. It appears that she was texting while driving, and that momentary distraction almost cost her life!

Obviously, Emily's story has nothing to do with Health. So, why am I talking about this? I am discussing this because, while health problems like high blood pressure can reduce your lifespan over time, distracted driving can cause you to lose life and limb in a matter of seconds. Living long is not just about physical health, but also a whole lot more including managing your dangerous habits.

The strength of a chain is at its weakest link. It does not matter how strong the rest of the chain is, it will always fail at the weakest link. That weak link in your case can be a health condition, a bad habit, an addiction, or a mental condition like depression. It makes sense to take an all-round 360-degree view of your life, identify the weak links, manage them and reduce your overall risks in a comprehensive manner. I cannot stress the word 'comprehensive' enough, because even if you ignore one problem out of many, that one problem can come back to haunt you!

IDENTIFYING THE WEAK LINKS

Now that we have made the point about weak links, let us focus on identifying and addressing them. This chapter is not about making lifestyle changes or other long term improvements. It is about identifying the specific problems that can potentially cause damage to you, and addressing each problem immediately in a focused manner, so that it stops being a risk to your health and wellness.

To be comprehensive, we need to address several Categories of potential weaknesses, as listed below:

- Physical health issues
- Mental health issues
- Fitness problems
- Bad habits
- Relaxation & sleep issues
- Relationship issues
- Other wellness issues

I have used an example of a middle-aged man for making this list below. His name is Joe, and he is not real. I invented Joe so that we can use him to illustrate how to use this chapter to your advantage.

Based on the categories listed above, let us fill the table below with the weak links or 'issues' that Joe has. The first column shows the category of the issue. The second column shows the specific issue Joe is suffering from. The third column shows the status of the issue.

The 'Status' column shows whether each issue is in control or not. It is important to note that some issues may not be in control even if Joe is taking medications or taking other actions to manage that issue.

The column 'Status' is important because, we want to pay attention to those issues that are not in control and bring them under control before they cause lasting damage. For example, high blood pressure that is not in control can cause continuous and irreversible damage to your body, and can lead to heart attack, kidney failure, stroke, dementia or any number of other serious problems:

Category	Issue	Status
Physical Health	High Blood Pressure	Not in control
	High Cholesterol	In control
	Acid Reflux	Not in control
Fitness	Overweight	Not in control
	Persistent lower back	In control
	Get tired too easily	In control
Bad habits	Texting while driving	Not in control
	Excessive alcohol consumption	Not in control
	Occasional smoking	In control
Relaxation & sleep	Insomnia	Not in control

Category	Issue	Status
	Highly stressful work conditions	In control
Mental Health	Depression	In control
Relationships	Going through divorce	Not in control
Other wellness issues	Too many loans	In control

By reviewing the list above, it appears that Joe has seven issues that are our of control, and need to be managed immediately. Let us how we can bring them under control in the next chapter.

MY ACTION ITEMS

Here are my action items from this chapter:
I have identified all the issues that can impact my health, wellness and longevity based on the categories listed above.

- If I have other issues belonging to categories not listed here, I have included them in the list.
- I have identified the issues that are 'Out of Control' now.
- I understand that the 'Out of Control' issues need immediate attention.
- I am willing to seek help from my primary care doctors or other experts as needed, to address my 'Out of Control' issues immediately.

I am ready for the next chapter.

Chapter 5
MANAGING THE CONDITIONS THAT ARE OUT OF CONTROL

Once you identify the chronic conditions that are out of control, it is necessary to seek professional help and bring those conditions quickly under control. Effective control of chronic conditions reduces your risks and increases your lifespan significantly.

In the previous chapter, we listed all the health and wellness issues for hypothetical Joe. We identified several of those issues as 'Out of Control'. Here is the list of issues that are out of control for Joe:

- High Blood Pressure
- Acid reflux
- Overweight
- Texting while driving
- Excessive Alcohol consumption
- Insomnia
- Going through divorce

This still looks like a long list. But if you look at this carefully, you may find that often, the things that go out of control are related to each other. Some of them may even have a cause and effect relationship, in the sense that some of the issues may be causing some of the other issues.

For example, in this case, if you can address the overweight issue and the excessive alcohol consumption issue, there is a chance that the High Blood Pressure issue may reduce. If you address the stress arising from the Divorce issue, you may be able to bring the insomnia issue under control. Obviously, these results are not guaranteed, but potentially possible. Therefore, it is important to list out all the known issues holistically.

For each of these issues above, there is a short-term intervention and a long-term solution. The short-term intervention is very important because these out-of-control issues are already causing damage every single day they remain out of control. It is important to bring these issues quickly under control so that they stop causing damage. The short-term intervention is what this chapter is about. The long-term solution follows in later chapters.

Intervention is best achieved by seeking professional help quickly. The professionals you consult have the right expertise to come up with a comprehensive plan and a timeline with you to address the issues. For example, when you see your primary care doctor regarding the uncontrolled high blood pressure, he or she may use a comprehensive method as follows:

- Conduct further diagnostics to look for root causes if any
- Prescribe or increase your medication
- Change the timing of your medication

- Increase the number of consultations until the condition gets under control
- Recommend weight reduction
- Recommend dietary changes and reduced sodium intake
- Recommend reduction of alcohol consumption
- Provide stress management guidelines and prescribe sleep medication
-

Seek help for excessive alcohol addiction. Dangerous habits like texting while driving need to be addressed immediately, and if you cannot address them on your own, share the problems with a family member, do whatever it takes to get rid of your dangerous habits. Seek professional help if needed.

Basically, leave it to the experts, follow their advice and work with them. Your main job is to keep seeking attention from these experts until you get all your out-of-control issues under control quickly and effectively.

Once you start this exercise, you should aim to get all the uncontrolled issues under good control within two to six weeks. Some issues may take more time, but having clear deadlines is a good way to accomplish targets.

After you get your issues under control, run this exercise every 12 months or more frequently. Learn how to list the issues out of control at that time, and bring them under control quickly. Keep in mind that things are changing all the time.

Keep in mind that your 'out of control' issues become your weak links, and sometimes even a single weak link can bring you down. It is necessary to bring all 'out of control' issues under control quickly.

It is likely that once you get all your issues under control, you may end up with several medications and other tedious routines every day. This is Ok for now. The next chapter will help reduce your dependence on medications and other tedious routines in partnership with the professionals you are already working with.

Do not reduce or stop taking your medications on your own, or stop using your therapies without consulting your doctors or other specialists. Remember, health is a team game. Use your team of experts efficiently.

MY ACTION ITEMS

Now that you have finished this chapter, here are your action items:

- I have consulted professionals regarding my out-of-control conditions.
- I have come up with an action plan for each 'out of control' issue.
- I have a plan to periodically review my conditions and seek help as needed.
-

I am ready for the next step!

PREVENTION

Making smart life choices that can keep you younger, stay stronger and live longer.

Chapter 5
SETTING UP YOUR PREVENTION PLAN

Human bodies were not designed to become weak and sick as we get older. Nature designed us to be strong and purposeful to the last day of our lives. However, to enjoy that outcome, we need to make healthy choices and lead active lives. This chapter is about a comprehensive overhaul of your lifestyle so that you can stay strong and live long.

In the previous chapters, we talked about intervention, which is mostly about identifying the health issues that are likely to make you weak, and addressing them so that they do not cause ongoing damage. In contrast, prevention is about making holistic lifestyle improvements that provide your body with the strength and immunity it needs, so that it can prevent disease and degeneration from happening in the first place. Prevention is always better than cure!

Your prevention plan is built around five main areas of lifestyle improvements. To strengthen your immunity and remain healthy to a ripe old age, you need to achieve and sustain optimal improvements in each of these five areas below:

- Weight management
- Nutrition
- Cardiovascular endurance
- Muscular strength, endurance and flexibility
- Relaxation

WHY MOST PREVENTION PLANS ARE NOT SUSTAINABLE

The lifestyle improvement areas listed above are well known to all of us. Almost everyone tries out various diets, exercise plans, and relaxation therapies over their lifetimes. Yet, majority of the people cannot sustain their plans, and give up over time. Some people try multiple times only to give up repeatedly and become cynical over time. Why is this?

There are five important reasons why lifestyle improvement plans fail, and here they are:

- **Not having a why:** Tony Robbins once said, if you want to accomplish anything of value, you need to understand your 'why' before you need to know your 'how'. In other words, if you do not have a strong enough reason for doing something, you will not be able to stick to doing it when the going gets tough.
- **Not having clear goals:** If you do not have clear goals, you will not know where you are in your journey and where you are going. It is easy to lose track this way.
- **Not using the right tools:** This is the most important reason why lifestyle plans fail. Not using the right tools can make the difference between sticking to a plan or not in the long run.

- **Not interesting:** Your plan should consist of things that are interesting, practical, addictive and fun for you to do. It should not consist of things you force yourself to do. Anything you force yourself to do cannot be sustained over a long time.
- **No check-and-adjust mechanism:** Every plan needs to be validated with reality and adjusted over time on a regular basis. If your plan does not involve a good process to check and adjust over time, it will not survive.

YOUR UNFAILING PLAN FOR LASTING HEALTH AND WELLNESS

Now that we know the five reasons why most plans fail, let me introduce you to a time-tested five step process to create a bullet proof plan for lasting health and wellness:

The five-step process:

Step 1: Understand your why	To stick to your prevention plan, you need to be clear about why you are interested in that plan in the first place. This should not be a superficial answer. Look deep!
Step 2: Set clear goals	We talked about five areas above that need to be improved to develop your strength and immunity. You need to set clear
Step 3: Select the right tools and accessories	This is obvious. Nothing works without using the right tools.

Step 4: Keep it interesting	Your plan should be built around things that are natural to you based on your choices, passions and beliefs. It should be easy, interesting, enjoyable, addicting, rewarding and convenient. It should not consist of things you should force yourself to do.
Step 5: Check and adjust	Once you launch the plan, you need to periodically check and adjust the areas that are not working optimally. Have patience. After you adjust your plan a few times, your plan will be working like a well-oiled machine!

In the next chapters, we will dive into each of these five steps in the sequence listed above.

Chapter 6
UNDERSTANDING YOUR WHY

We have heard of stories where someone hung on to life against medical odds until a relative or friend arrived at their bedside, or until a special anniversary or birthday. This is not unusual. There is ample proof that people with a strong purpose tend to live longer and stay healthier.

The Japanese who live on the island of Okinawa are one of the longest-lived people in the world. Okinawa is one of the longevity zones discovered by Dan Buettner, the founder of the Blue Zones project. One of the factors in Okinawan's longevity is what they call ikigai. This word means "the reason for being" or the purpose of your life.

Yes, we all have a purpose to be strong, healthy, successful, and wealthy. But these are superficial purposes. The word "ikigai" is used to refer to a deeper purpose. Why do you want to be strong, healthy, successful, and wealthy? What's your larger purpose? How can you impact the world and leave it better than you found it?

Finding your ikigai or purpose is the key to living a fulfilling life. Once you know your purpose and begin to fulfill it, you feel that your life is complete. Then nothing can faze you. You have the courage to face any challenge, endure any loss or setback, and keep striving no matter what. It frees you from lesser desires that can sidetrack you away from your purpose.

Okinawans have found their purpose/ikigai. This knowledge is with them when they wake up every morning, and they are excited and ready to fulfill it. They understand that their ikigai isn't about doing something that's selfish or self-centered but about giving back. By finding their ikigai, they have the added benefit of adding seven years to their lives, as discovered by the Blue Zones team.

To make your prevention plan sustainable, you need to find your ikigai. You need to understand why you want to live long and stay healthy and how the world is going to be different because of it. You need to be able to visualize the impact you can make.

What does being healthy and fit mean for you and the world? Why is this important?

Maybe you like the prospect of traveling and seeing places, hiking your next mountain and motivating other people to follow an active lifestyle. Maybe you like to spend more time with your family. Maybe you like spoiling your grandchildren with gifts and hugs. Or maybe you're the kind of person who likes to volunteer, give back, build parks for needy kids. To do all these things, you need to be healthy and strong. The longer you live, the more you can give back!

Whatever your reasons are for seeking a healthier and longer life, feel it and visualize it. Imagine those mountains you'll be climbing. Imagine those lives you'll be impacting. Understand your why! This helps you to keep going and stay steadfast to your goals when the going gets tough.

MY ACTION ITEMS

To find your ikigai, answer the following four questions:

- What do I love to do?
- What am I good at doing?
- How can I positively impact the world?
- How can I get paid to fulfill my ikigai?

When you finally find your ikigai, you'll discover that the universe opens in magnificent ways and supports you in your mission. Give and you shall receive!

Chapter 7
SETTING UP YOUR GOALS

The first step towards making successful lifestyle improvements is to have clear goals that are simple, measurable, achievable, relevant and time-bound (SMART)

Now that you've discovered your ikigai in the previous chapter, we'll move on to setting up holistic goals for your prevention plan. We'll cover the following five areas as discussed before:

- Weight management goals
- Nutrition goals
- Cardiovascular endurance goals
- Muscular strength, endurance and flexibility goals
- Rest and relaxation goals

WEIGHT MANAGEMENT GOALS

In simple terms, weight Management is the practice of attaining and maintaining an optimal body weight by balancing a healthy diet with physical activity.

Why weight management is important
Out of all the things you can do for your health, weight management is among the most important because it has a cascading effect on every other aspect of your health and longevity. Also, it's a tangible goal which is easy to measure and monitor.

When weight isn't managed well, it becomes the single most negative factor in impacting your lifespan. Being overweight increases the risk of several health problems, including heart disease, diabetes, hypertension and kidney problems. Excess weight in pregnant women may lead to long-term and short-term health problems for both mother and child.

Several kinds of health problems are linked to being overweight. Here's a partial list:

- High blood pressure
- Heart disease
- Strokes
- Acid reflux
- Type 2 diabetes
- Kidney disease
- Certain types of cancer
- Sleep apnea
- Osteoarthritis
- Fatty liver disease
-

How about being underweight?
Being underweight also carries several health risks as follows:

- Malnutrition, anemia, vitamin deficiencies
- Decreased immune function
- Osteoporosis from too little Vitamin D and Calcium

- Increased risk of complications from surgery
- Growth and development issues, especially in children

Why getting to ideal weight makes the greatest difference!

When an overweight or underweight person gets back to normal weight, the impacts to health are not only substantial but also almost instantaneous. Here are some examples where you can feel the impact of weight management very quickly:

High Blood Pressure: Blood pressure is how hard your blood pushes against the walls of your arteries as it pumps though your blood vessels to the rest of your body. A blood pressure of 120/80 mm Hg is considered normal. If your higher number is above 140, or lower the number is above 90, then your blood pressure is considered high. High blood pressure is linked to heart attack, heart disease, stroke, kidney disease, dementia, and a host of other problems.

High blood pressure is linked to obesity and excess weight. If you're overweight and have high blood pressure, a small drop of 10% weight can bring your hypertension under control and reduce the need for medication. This reduction in Blood Pressure can be seen immediately, as soon as you reduce weight!

Type 2 Diabetes: This is a disease in which blood sugar levels are above normal. High blood sugar is a major cause of kidney disease, stroke, heart disease, blindness, amputations, and a host of other conditions. Being overweight increases the likelihood of developing type 2 diabetes.

One of the reasons is that the excess weight reduces our body's sensitivity to a hormone called Insulin, which, in turn, reduces the body's ability to use the sugar being delivered by blood to various organs of the body. Clinical studies have shown that just dropping 5 to 10% of body weight coupled with moderate exercise can prevent or delay the onset of type 2 diabetes!

This is just a short and partial list of advantages from weight loss. But it's enough to show us that getting back to ideal weight has very powerful and lasting advantages for your health and well-being.

What's my ideal weight?
There are several ways to find your ideal weight. Here's one of the simplest means of calculating your ideal weight:

- Go to the website: https://www.calculator.net/ ideal-weight-calculator.html
- Plug in your age, gender, and height.
- Click the "Calculate" button. The calculator produces four different "Ideal Weight" numbers based on four different formulas. It also provides an ideal weight range.

Let's use an example for this chapter. Let's say you're a 44-year-old male, with a height of 5 feet and 10 inches. By putting those numbers into the calculator above, you get your ideal body weight to be the following four choices based on four different formulas:

1. Robinson formula: 156.5 pounds
2. Miller formula: 155 pounds
3. Devine: 160.9 pounds
4. Hamwi: 165.3 pounds

The results also show that any weight between 128.9 and 174.2 pounds is in the healthy range. You can see that there's a wide variation in these four numbers. I usually consider the lowest of the four numbers, which is 155 pounds in this case, to be my ideal weight.

How much weight do I have to lose or gain to get to my ideal weight?

Using the example above, if your current weight is 200 pounds, then you must lose 45 pounds to get to your ideal weight of 155 pounds. If you're underweight at 120 pounds, then you must gain 35 pounds to get to your ideal weight.

How long do I have to get to my ideal weight?

If you want to be aggressive and you're generally healthy, you can lose up to two pounds every week safely. However, it's better to be more gradual. Losing one pound per week is more sustainable. If you have any preexisting health conditions, make sure you talk to your doctor before you start altering your weight drastically.

Your weight management goals summary

Based on the example numbers we're using above, here are your numbers:

Your current weight: 200 pounds
Your ideal weight (goal weight): 155 pounds
Weight loss needed to get to ideal weight: 45 pounds
Duration for weight loss (at one pound per week): 45 weeks

Now that we have our S.M.A.R.T goals for weight management, let's move on to our next goal.

NUTRITION GOALS

In this section, we'll work about setting up your nutrition goals.

Good nutrition is a critical part of leading a healthy lifestyle. When combined with physical activity, your nutrition plan can help you to reach and maintain a healthy weight, reduce your risk of chronic diseases like heart disease and cancer, and promote your overall health.

We'll start with some ground rules:

Ground rules for a sustainable nutrition plan

Rule 1: Regardless of which diet plan you may choose to follow, it should involve these seven natural food groups: fruits, vegetables, whole grains, legumes, nuts, dairy, and lean protein sources.

Rule 2: Your plan should avoid or reduce junk food, defined as food that's low in nutrients, high in calories, and may contain chemical additives. Here are some types of junk food you should avoid:

- Refined carbohydrates - like white rice, pasta, pastries, cookies, cakes, white bread
- Sugary food - like carbonated beverages, ice creams, fruit juices, etc.
- Highly processed junk foods - like nitrate-treated meats and packaged food like microwave popcorn, breakfast cereals, and canned soup.
- Fried foods - like French fries and potato chips
- High calorie foods - like Pizza

Rule 3: Your plan should include all seven macro-nutrients required for the human body: fats, protein, carbohydrates, fiber, vitamins, minerals, and water.

Rule 4: Your nutrition plan shouldn't be something dictated by a diet plan that someone else set in place. It should consist of food that you love to eat, practical and easy to find based on your specific circumstances.

If you follow these ground rules, you'll end up selecting a nutrition plan that's customized for you based on your preferences, ease, and practicality and affordability of following it.

The secret of a good nutrition plan is that it shouldn't take a lot of determination and will power to stay on the plan. It should consist of foods you enjoy and crave. It should be addictive, practical and easy to follow.

Okay, it's time to move on to the next step. Before we make our diet choices, let's start with reviewing some of the popular diet-plans we have all heard of.

Brief review of diet plans out-there

We will review some popular diet plans briefly, as a prerequisite for our nutrition planning. There are literally hundreds of diet-plans available. Someone comes up with a new one almost every week. Here is the list:

- Mediterranean Diet
- Vegan Diet
- Paleo Diet
- Low Carb Diets
- Atkins Diet
- Zone Diet

Let's analyze these diet plans and review some of their upsides and downsides.

Mediterranean Diet: Interest in this diet grew around the 1960s because of its association with reduced risk factors for cardiovascular disease. This diet is easy to follow because it's well balanced and doesn't eliminate any food group. One downside of Mediterranean diet is potential mercury ingestion because of fish consumption.

Vegan diet: The vegan diet prescribes food coming from purely plant sources. It restricts animal products for ethical, environmental, or health reasons, and eliminates meat, dairy, eggs, and animal-derived products such as gelatin, honey, albumin, whey, and casein.

Plant-based diets are linked to a reduced risk of heart disease and type 2 diabetes, Alzheimer's, and cancer. On the downside, vegan diets may be low in some nutrients, including vitamin B12, vitamin D, iodine, omega-3 fatty acids, iron, calcium, and zinc. This means that some supplementation or an additional balancing act is required.

Paleo Diet: The paleo diet prescribes the same foods that our hunter-gatherer ancestors ate before farming was developed. The theory is that most modern diseases are linked to eating diary, grains, and processed foods. Basically, this diet emphasizes whole foods, vegetables, lean protein, fruits, nuts, and seeds, while reducing or eliminating the intake of processed foods, sugar, dairy, and grains.

Studies have shown that the paleo diet is effective in maintaining a healthy weight and reducing risk factors for heart disease such as cholesterol, blood sugar, triglycerides, and high blood pressure. The downside is that this diet eliminates whole grains, dairy, and legumes, which are nutritious and healthy.

Low-Carb Diets: Low-carb diets have been popular for a long time, especially for weight loss. They emphasize unlimited amounts of protein and fat while severely limiting your carb intake. The primary aim of the diet is to force your body to use more fats for fuel instead of using carbs as a main source of energy. Low-carbs diets are affective because they reduce your craving for food.

They may also help with many major disease risk factors such as blood triglycerides, blood pressure, cholesterol, blood sugar, and insulin levels. The downside is that low-carb diets don't suit everyone, especially those who are vegetarian or vegan. Some feel great while others feel miserable.

Atkins Diet: The Atkins diet is a popular version of the low-carb diet. It prescribes that you can lose weight by eating as much protein and fat as you like if you avoid carbs. The main reason why low-carb diets are effective for weight loss is that they reduce your appetite. They're especially successful in reducing belly fat, the most dangerous fat that lodges itself in your abdominal cavity. It's also known to reduce many risk factors for disease, including cholesterol, triglycerides, blood sugar, high blood pressure, and insulin.

The downside of the Atkins Diet is that it eliminates carbs some of which may be very healthy and nutritious. Also, high protein low carb diets rely on fatty cuts of meat, whole dairy products, and other high-fat foods that are likely raise cholesterol, increase your chance of heart disease, kidney problems, osteoporosis and kidney stones.

Zone Diet: The Zone diet prescribes a daily calorie combination of about 30% fat, 30% protein and 40% carbohydrates. It further prescribes that the carbohydrates used should have low glycemic index (GI).

The Glycemic Index of a food is an estimate of how much it raises your blood glucose level after consumption. Basically, it recommends that the carbs should mostly come from colorful fruits, veggies, and whole grains. It recommends avoiding high glycemic carbs like bananas, rice, and potatoes.

Benefits of this diet include reduction in risk factors like high blood pressure, cholesterol, and triglycerides, and a reduction in food-induced inflammation and waist size. As a drawback, this diet limits the consumption of some healthy carb sources, such as bananas and potatoes.

What should your diet plan look like?

Based on the brief review of the different diet plans above, which ones did you like? I personally like the Mediterranean diet. I don't like the low-carb diets because, being vegetarian, low-carb diets don't work very well for me. Your choices may be different from mine.

However, I don't like being restricted to Mediterranean or any specific type of diet. Let's go a little bit deeper into this, okay? The reason I like Mediterranean isn't because it's a specific type of diet I'm into, but rather because it's a balanced and natural diet with plenty of fruits, vegetables, grains, nuts, seeds, lean protein sources, diary, olive oil, and wine. But I would also like to eat a wide variety of other diets like Indian, Asian, American, Italian, Mexican, Vietnamese, and good old

American. I like all kinds of food and I don't like being restricted to Mediterranean alone.

Also, I don't like the other inconveniences that come with following specific diet plans. I do not like restricting my grocery shopping to only certain kinds of food, cooking only certain kinds of meals, going to only certain kinds of restaurants that offer the kind of food I can eat, and so on.

If I'm on a specific diet plan, I know I will always crave those other forbidden foods that are not part of my diet. This situation is even worse if you follow an extreme diet like high protein diet. Your food choices become extremely limited. I don't like these restrictions at all. I don't like any plan that requires me to exercise my will power and determination to stick to it. Such plans aren't sustainable.

If you want to stick to a diet plan over your lifetime, it cannot be built around restrictions, discipline, and denial. It shouldn't require you to exercise determination and will-power. It shouldn't call for sacrifices. It should allow you to enjoy a wide variety of choices that you love, while keeping you healthy. This is where the four ground rules I listed above come in handy.

Let's run a quick exercise to see how you can use the four ground rules to build the best diet plan for yourself, one that you can follow for the rest of your life. We'll call this the "Practical plan." I'll use myself as the subject. The plan I'm about to show you is specific to me, and it will look different when you make your plan. But that's the whole point!

I'll start with listing out the meals that I love to eat, meals that are convenient and practical for me.

I live in a suburb. I must get up early in the morning and go to work in a bustling city. Before I go to work, I have my breakfast at home.

I start my breakfast with a strong cup of coffee, with added cream and honey.

Here are the breakfast choices I love and find convenient and practical:

- Egg omelet with vegetables and cheese.
- Triple berries smoothie with whey protein and almonds.
- Paleo power bar with nuts and seeds.
- Black bean burger patty with a small orange.
- Scrambled eggs and cheese and a side fruit salad
- One egg waffle with a small orange

As I said above, I work in a bustling city. I like to eat out during lunch. I have many great choices for lunch. Here are my preferred lunch choices:

- Jimmy John's sandwich with extra veggies, avocado and cheese
- Subway sandwich with veggie patty
- Salad with mixed greens, oranges, dried cranberries, avocado and candied pecans.
- Black bean curry with white rice, with a cup of Pepsi
- Spinach curry with white rice, with a cup of Pepsi
- Falafel sandwich with hummus
- Two tacos with coleslaw and cheese, with a small side order of rice and beans
- Veggie patty sandwich with French fries
- Thai curry with rice
- Small pizza with veggie toppings

Here are some afternoon snacks I was used to:

- Bag of Doritos chips
- Bag of spicy potato chips
- Cookie

I go home in the evening and usually have a sumptuous homemade meal or a take-out dinner and relax with my family. I always start with two glasses of red wine and unwind from my day before starting on my dinner. Here are my favorite dinner choices:

- Brown rice with veggie curry followed by high-protein Chobani yogurt with brown rice
- Pasta with bread and a small house salad
- Ravioli with bread and a small house salad
- Cheese enchilada with rice and beans
- Two veggie tacos with rice and beans
- Falafel sandwich with hummus
- Lasagna with bread

Again, I want to remind you that these are my preferences based on what I love and what's practical and easy for me. This is my reality. You can make your own list with your personal preferences!

Now that we have the list of food choices, let's validate this list against the four ground rules we came up with earlier.

- **Rule 1:** If you see the list of my choices, you can see that they consist of a liberal mix of fruits, vegetables, whole grains, legumes, nuts, dairy and lean protein sources. Rule 1 is satisfied.

- **Rule 2:** Upon reviewing the choices, we do find that there's some junk food in that mix. There are some choices of Pepsi and white rice. I can avoid Pepsi altogether, and replace white rice with brown rice. I can replace my afternoon snack choices which are mostly chips and cookies, with hummus dip and celery, or just get rid of the afternoon snacks. With these minimal changes, I can satisfy Rule 2.

- **Rule 3:** The list of my food choices above does contain all the nutrients needed by human bodies, fats, protein, carbohydrates, fiber, vitamins, minerals, and water. To validate this rule, we will need a diet management App that can evaluate the nutrition content of most foods we normally eat. We can validate that later when we discuss tools and artifacts. Rule 3 is satisfied.

- **Rule 4:** My food choices above are based on my personal preferences. I love these foods and I'm addicted to them. These are also practical choices, since I have been already using them and they're easy to find near my home or office. Rule 4 is satisfied.

This is it. Take a good look at the food choices I ended up with. Does it look like I'm following any kind of restrictive diet? I feel like I'm having a feast every day. My daily diet consists of things I love and crave to eat. It also satisfies the four ground rules we've listed above toward ensuring that my diet is healthy and sustainable over a long time.

This is how you create a diet plan you can stick to for life!

CARDIOVASCULAR ENDURANCE GOALS

You finished working on your weight management and nutrition goals. The next step is to work on your cardiovascular endurance goal. So, what does this term mean?

Cardiovascular endurance is your body's ability to keep up with activities like hiking, running, jogging, swimming, and cycling that force your lungs, heart, and blood vessels to work under pressure for extended periods of time. Together, the heart and lungs fuel your body with the oxygen needed by your muscles for the work they're doing.

How can you tell if you have good cardiovascular endurance? It's easy. You'll be out of breath walking a few city blocks or climbing a few flights of stairs if your cardiovascular endurance isn't good. This is because your heart and lungs aren't providing the necessary oxygen in an efficient manner to perform the work your body is doing.

Increasing your cardiovascular endurance is an important step toward maintaining your health, fitness, and vitality for life. By improving your cardiovascular endurance, you can avoid health problems like the ones below:

- High blood pressure
- Heart attack
- Heart failure
- Type II diabetes
- Elevated cholesterol
- Coronary heart disease
- Hardening of blood vessels

Your cardiovascular endurance goal

Numerous aerobic activities, such as walking, jogging, running, hiking, aerobics, cycling, swimming, rowing, stair climbing, cross country skiing, and dancing, can increase your cardiovascular endurance. Sports, such as basketball, tennis, soccer, and squash, can also improve your cardiovascular fitness.

Personally, I like walking, hiking, and jogging. This is because these activities are easy to track. They can be performed indoors on a treadmill or outdoors in a wide variety of environments. They don't require special gear other than a good pair of shoes and clothing that's appropriate for the weather.

As a guideline, if you're generally healthy, taking 10,000 steps a day is considered a good cardiovascular endurance goal. It burns about 500 calories, covers an average of five miles and takes roughly 90 minutes of brisk walking.

You don't have to do all these steps in one chunk. You should walk throughout the day as part of your normal activities anyway. If you can meet a cumulative goal of 10,000 steps by adding all your steps throughout the day, it's okay. This isn't such a hard goal to achieve every day.

If you're interested in other activities besides walking, just make sure you're burning an equivalent of 500 calories as part of your daily goal. It doesn't matter what activity you're involved in if you're meeting the calorie goal.

In addition to spending the calories, it's also beneficial to raise your heart rate when you're performing your aerobic activity. Generally, cardio gains are optimal if you increase your heart rate from 50% to 85% of your highest heart rate. To come up with this number, subtract your age from the number 220. Let's say if you're fifty-five years old, then your target heart rate while performing your aerobic routine is (220 - 55), which is 165.

How do you know that you're improving your cardiovascular endurance?
Let's say you're keeping up with your cardiovascular goals, the best way to know if you're making improvements is to test it periodically. There are two popular tests, which are fairly accurate:

- **The Cooper run:** This test measures the maximum distance you can run in 12 minutes. The longer the distance you can cover, the more your endurance.

- **The step test:** This test makes you step up and down on an aerobics-type pedestal for five minutes to increase heart rate, and then evaluates how long it takes for your heart to return to normal rate immediately following the test. The sooner it gets back to normal, the better off you are.

Aerobic endurance is a very important indicator of health and longevity. Make sure this is part of your daily routine.

It is now time to move on to the next goal.

MUSCULAR STRENGTH, ENDURANCE, AND FLEXIBILITY GOALS

Now that you're done setting up your cardio goals, let's work on setting up your muscular fitness goals.

Your muscles help you perform all the daily activities needed, including utilitarian movements, lifting and moving weights, and protecting your body. To perform these activities, they need strength, endurance, and flexibility, which are three different aspects of muscular fitness.

Muscular strength is the amount of weight your muscles can lift. Without muscular strength, your body would be weak and unable to keep up with the demands placed upon it.

Muscular endurance is how many times you can move that weight without getting exhausted or very tired. Basically, endurance is the ability of your muscles to perform contractions for extended periods of time.

Muscular flexibility is the ability to bend and flex so that your body has the maximum possible range of movement. Without flexibility, the muscles and joints would grow stiff and movement would be limited.

Why are muscular strength, endurance and flexibility important?
Muscular strength is important because:

- It increases your ability to perform daily activities like lifting weights.
- Helps maintain a healthier body while reducing the risk of injury.
- Increases your confidence and your sense of accomplishment.
- Burns more calories while resting and helps maintain a healthy body weight.
- Helps maintain stronger bones.

Muscular endurance is important because:

- You can sustain your ability to perform an activity for a longer duration.
- Helps get through the day performing more activities without getting tired.

Muscular flexibility is important because:

- It ensures that your body can move through its entire range of motion without pain or stiffness.
- It helps with injury prevention.
- It contributes to avoiding conditions like arthritis and more serious illnesses.
- It reduces the risk of cardiovascular disease.
- Reduces stiffness in the arterial walls, an indicator of the risk for stroke and heart attack.

How do I improve muscular strength, endurance, and flexibility?
Weight training is required to improve strength and endurance. Flexibility can be increased by performing stretching exercises. Generally, strength training focuses on lifting heavier weights with fewer sets and repetitions, whereas endurance exercises require lesser weights with more sets and repetitions.

You can start your muscular fitness journey by answering a few simple questions regarding your preferences:

- Are you planning to build muscles or just keep in good shape?
- How often are you planning to visit the gym? Every day? Every other day?
- How much time can you spend in the gym every time you go?
- Can you invest in personal or group training?
- Are you in good health?

- Do you have any preexisting conditions that can impact your ability to lift weights and stretch?

To optimize your weight training and stretching outcomes, it's necessary that you learn how to perform the exercises in the right way and avoid injury. It's best to discuss your preferences with a personal trainer, and get that person to come up with a plan for increasing your strength, endurance, and flexibility in a holistic and sustainable manner. Once you have the plan, have that person show you the correct way of performing those exercises.

Some people end up buying exercise equipment so that they can workout at home. I generally discourage this approach. Maintaining optimal muscle fitness requires exercising with a wide variety of equipment, often altering the weights and range of motion. Unless you're willing to invest in a lot of equipment and weights, it's preferable to have someone else invest in all that and just go to a gym. Besides, you can meet personal trainers in a gym, which is harder to do at home.

How do I know if I'm improving?
If you're regularly exercising and staying active, you'll notice that your ability to lift weights is improving, and your ability to perform more sets and reps with the same weights is improving as well. In addition, regularly working out increases your body tone and makes you look more ripped and stronger. It's not hard to notice these changes.

To make your muscular fitness goals viable and sustainable, it's necessary to select a gym that's near to your home or work and develop a habit of visiting it regularly. This is where most people fail. They start with enthusiasm and keep paying their monthly dues but don't go to the health club as often as they should.

Work out with a partner or a friend who can keep you motivated. Engage a trainer who can keep you true to your goal. Sign up for group fitness activities that can keep you motivated. Relax in the Jacuzzi or swimming pool at the gym after working out so that you're motivated to go more often. Keep it interesting.

Now that you understand how to set your goals for muscular fitness, let's move on to the next section.

REST AND RELAXATION GOALS

You're now in the final stretch of setting your goals.

Rest and relaxation often don't get the attention they deserve. Your daily activities break down your body and make you tired. After a hard day of work, it's necessary for you to unwind, relax, and get a good night's sleep. During this down-time, your body repairs, rejuvenates, and rebuilds itself, and the mind resets for a fresh new start the next day. It's easy for your health to deteriorate if you're not getting enough rest.

Rest, relaxation, and good sleep have numerous advantages. Here are a few:

- Better concentration and improved productivity
- Reduced risk of weight gain
- Greater athletic performance
- Lower risk of heart disease
- Improved social and emotional intelligence
- Stronger immune system

Here are some disadvantages of not getting enough rest and sleep:

- Increased susceptibility to accidents
- Reduced sharpness of your mind
- Increased potential of illness including heart disease, stroke, and diabetes
- Depression
- Accelerated aging
- Forgetfulness
- Weight gain

Obviously, it's important to address any roadblocks to getting enough rest and sleep. To do so, you should first understand the causes of losing sleep.

What causes lack of rest and sleep?
Here are some important reasons for not getting enough rest and sleep:

- Stress due to work, finances, relationships, career, health, etc.
- Travel across multiple time zones, working during late, early, or changing shifts
- Poor sleep environment and habits
- Eating too much in the evening
- Mental health disorders
- Medications
- Caffeine, alcohol, and nicotine

If you're not getting enough rest and sleep, you should look for the reasons above and address them effectively. If necessary, get professional help in addressing them.

How do you measure the quality of your rest and sleep?
Sleep quality is measured by several parameters such as total duration of sleep, duration of deep sleep, duration

and intensity of snoring or sleep apnea, and the feeling of restfulness and energy when you wake up.

While many of these attributes appear to be quite subjective, many devices and apps can measure your sleep quality well. By measuring regularly, you increase your ability to improve it. We'll discuss the various apps and devices in the next chapter.

Goals for restful sleep
Here are some goals for restful sleep:

- Getting at least 6 to 8 hours of sleep
- At least 2 hours of deep sleep
- No snoring
- Feeling of well-rested freshness when you get up in the morning

Congratulations! You've finished a long chapter dedicated to setting your goals. Now, let's quickly go through your checklist of action items.

MY ACTION ITEMS

Here are the action items for this chapter:

- I have set my weight management goal.
- I have understood the four ground rules for good nutrition.
- I have reviewed the various popular diet goals.
- I have set my nutrition goal.
- I have set my cardiovascular endurance goal.
- I have set my muscular strength, endurance, and flexibility goals.
- I have set my rest and relaxation goal.

Chapter 8
USING THE RIGHT TOOLS AND ACCESSORIES

We are not the strongest of the species, the tallest, the heaviest, the fiercest or the most resilient. We do not have sharp claws. We do not have thick skins that can withstand extreme temperatures. And yet, we have scaled the tallest mountains, survived the most extreme temperatures, reached the depths of oceans, and reached out into space. The only way we could overcome our limitations and accomplish all these feats is by using the amazing tools and accessories we have invented.

In the previous chapters, we went through a detailed goal-setting process. In this chapter, we will explore how to use the right tools and accessories to make those goals practical and easy to pursue.

Specifically, we will set up some tools and accessories for managing the following goals:

- Weight management goals
- Nutrition goals

- Cardiovascular endurance goals
- Muscular strength, endurance and flexibility goals
- Rest and relaxation goals

TOOLS FOR WEIGHT MANAGEMENT

You may have heard the saying "What gets tracked gets improved". To change anything for the better, you need to know where you are and how far you need to go. Tracking your weight is an important part of getting to ideal weight and maintaining it.

The best way to track your weight is by using a smart scale. In addition to measuring your weight, smart scales these days can measure your body fat, water content, muscle mass, bone mass, BMI, BMR and other statistics. They can also relay the measurements over Bluetooth to an App on your smartphone.

The app can then not only store your measurements over time, it can flag those measurements as low, normal or high, so you know how your health stats compare to what's considered standard in health and fitness for your height and age!

Here are some of the popular smart scales in the market as of the date of writing this book. You cannot go wrong with any of these:

- Eufy smart scale
- Withings body cardio
- Runners-up Garmin index
- Fitbit aria 2
- Weight watchers smart scale

Tracking your weight every day gives you an early warning when you are deviating away from your ideal weight, and helps you get back on track before it is too late to do so. Especially around the holidays when we tend to gain weight, tracking it every day sets off a daily awareness in your mind to watch what you are eating and stay responsible.

TOOLS FOR NUTRITION MANAGEMENT

While weight management is a simple concept, managing your daily nutrition can be very complex and tedious affair. Back in the old days, you had to manually keep track of various things like daily calories, nutrition and exercise to maintain and manage your weight. Luckily, today, we have some Apps on our smartphones that can make it all easy and give us enormous capabilities in managing our nutrition goals.

Selecting your right App for nutrition management
Here are some popular Apps for nutrition management:

- MyFitnessPal
- LoseIt
- SparkPeople
- FitBit
- Weightwatchers

I use MyFitnessPal every day. It is an incredible App nutrition database of over 5 million different foods. This even includes many restaurant and ethnic foods that are not always easy to track!

Setting up your goals in the App
Download the App on your cellphone and set up your account. Once your account is set up, there is some initial configuration necessary, as described below.

- Go to "More -> Goals".
- Here, you will find different areas to set up your weight loss, nutrition and fitness goals.
- Once you set up your weight loss goals, MyFitnessPal will calculate the number of calories you need to consume every day to sustain that weight loss.
- In the nutrition goals area, you can decide how to split the daily calories between your different meals. I usually split my calories into four equal parts for breakfast, lunch, afternoon snacks and dinner.
- In the nutrition goals area, you can also decide the macronutrient proportions that contribute to your daily calories. For example, you can decide that 30% of your calories should come from protein, 30% from fat, and 40% from carbohydrates.
- In the fitness goals, you can decide how often you want to work out per week and how many minutes you plan to spend every time you work out.

Once you set up these goals on a one-time basis, MyFitnessPal can start tracking your goals, send you timely reminders and provide you ongoing feedback on how well you are doing!

Setting up your meal choices, aerobic and workout routines on the App.
Once you configure the goals as described above, you can start tracking your daily nutrition and exercises without any further configuration. However, it still takes some effort to type the names of the foods you eat, and the exercise routines you follow. Instead, you can drastically reduce your manual typing by saving your meals and workout choices in the App.

For example, let us say you have a favorite salad for lunch that consists of greens, avocado, pecans, dried cranberries, and oranges, with sweet maple dressing. Obviously, there is no specific name for this salad, and therefore you cannot find it in your diet tracking app. However, let us say you save this as a Meal, with approximate serving sizes for each of the components, and give it a name. As you are entering each component, the App provides you calorie counts for the component based on the serving sizes you have selected.

Here is what that meal can look like.

Avocado Pecan Salad
Components:

1. Mixed greens (50 calories)
2. One scoop of avocado (80 calories)
3. One scoop of candied pecan (80 calories)
4. One scoop of peeled oranges (70 calories)
5. One serving of sweet maple dressing (120 calories)

TOTAL: (400 calories)

In addition to saving the number of calories for the meal, the App also saves the macro and micro nutrients in this meal. By saving your favorite meals in the App like this, you can save yourself the trouble of having to type in each component every time you track it. Over time, you can create a large menu of your favorite choices!

You should go ahead and save the Meal choices you made while setting your nutrition goals in the previous chapter.

Just like you can save your Meal choices, you can also save the exercise choices you made while setting your cardiovascular endurance, muscular strength, endurance and flexibility goals.

Tracking your daily diet and exercises

At this point, you are done configuring the App for your needs. The App is now ready to track your daily diet and exercises. Based on how well you have done the configuration, it should take no more than at total of sixty seconds for tracking your breakfast, lunch, snacks, dinner, aerobics, weights and stretching exercises each day. The App automatically tracks your daily calorie intake, the macro and micro nutrients for each day. This App can become an incredible ally for you to track your lifestyle and health for the rest of your life!

Adjusting your daily diet and exercises

This is probably the most important aspect of tracking your daily diet and exercises. Your App has several analytical reports that show you how well you are keeping up with the diet, nutrition, calorie and exercise goals you set for yourself over time. You can keep adjusting until you are meeting your goals on a consistent basis.

It is easy to tell daily whether you are staying within your calorie limits and getting sufficient exercises. It is not as easy to tell whether you are meeting your macronutrient goals. For me, being predominantly vegetarian, it was a challenge to meet my daily goal of Protein consumption and I was taking in too much carbohydrates.

But over time, based on the reports from my App, I could make smart choices with my diet to take in more Protein while remaining predominantly vegetarian. I could not have done this without the App.

ACCESSORIES FOR EXERCISING

While Apps can track a lot of your lifestyle actions, there are several accessories that can help as well. Here are some:

- Smart watches from Apple and android, or wearables from Fitbit, etc. can track your walking habits and calories burnt. They can also seamlessly upload this information to the App of your choice.
- Using the right shoes or sneakers based on where you walk can help keep you comfortable and motivated.
- Subscribing to a music streaming service on your smartphone can keep you motivated during your workouts. Research has shown that people who listen to music are more likely to exercise longer and remain more consistent.
- Wearing the right clothing based on the environment where you exercise can help you work out through the year regardless of weather and other conditions.

These are only a few accessories that can make your daily pursuit of a good lifestyle much easier. yes, it costs some money to acquire these as a one-time investment, but it is well worth the benefits.

TOOLS FOR TRACKING
YOUR SLEEP

If you are having severe sleep problems that is impacting your daily performance and health, you should see a doctor. However, if you are trying to just improve your sleep patterns on a consistent basis, there are several smartphone Apps that can help. While the Apps are not as accurate as conducting a sleep test in a clinical setting, they are inexpensive or free, easy to use, and are consistently available for ongoing improvement.

Selecting your right App for tracking sleep
Here are some popular Apps for tracking sleep:

- Sleep Cycle
- Good morning alarm clock
- MotionX 24/7
- Auto sleep

Here are some wearable devices that can track your sleep patterns as well:

- Apple watch
- Android watch
- Fitbit
- Beddit

This is certainly not an exhaustive list of Apps and wearable devices out there. New ones are coming to the market all the time. Some Apps can interact with multiple tracking devices over Bluetooth, and can collect sleep information from those devices.

I use Sleep Cycle for tracking my sleep patterns. This app is very easy to use. When you go to bed, just keep the phone on the nightstand, connect it to the charger and turn on the Sleep Cycle App. Once turned on, it tracks the quality of your sleep through the night.

When you wake up you can see the time you went to bed and woke up, the 'percentage' of restful sleep, the number of total sleep hours' vs the number of deep sleep hours, and how long you snored if you did.

If you are not getting roughly 6 hours of consistent sleep and at least 2 hours of deep sleep, or if you are snoring consistently, you should take corrective action. This corrective action can be in the form of self-analysis to understand what is causing the lack of sleep or snoring, and coming up with action items to help address those problems. If you are unsuccessful, then you should see a sleep specialist. Not getting good sleep can cause severe problems to your health and well-being.

This is it! You have finished setting up Tools and Accessories that can make your pursuit of fitness possible and practical. Great job! Now, let us move on to the next step.

MY ACTION ITEMS

Here are the action items for this chapter:

- I have selected a suitable smart scale based on available choices.
- I have configured the smart scale to integrate with my smartphone or online app.
- I have selected appropriate App(s) for nutrition and exercise management
- I have configured my goals for weight, nutrition 7 exercise on the App(s).
- I have configured my favorite meals, beverages and exercises on the App.
- I have procured suitable accessories to help with my daily exercising.
- I have set my cardiovascular endurance goal.
- I have selected an appropriate App for tracking my sleep.

I am ready for the next chapter!

Chapter 9
LAUNCHING AND TRACKING YOUR PLAN

When you are in the planning stage, spend enough time and be deliberate in making your plan detailed and thorough. Planning should be deliberate. But following the plan every day should be quick and easy. Any plan that is hard to use every day and takes too much time will not be sustainable in the long term.

So far, you have spent a significant amount of time and effort planning your goals, setting up your tools and your approach. Now, it is time to launch the plan and get it running every day. The best part of this is, if the planning was done well, it should take no more than three to five minutes a day to run the plan!

Based on your plan, here are your action items for each day:

DAILY ACTION ITEMS

Here are the daily action items based on your plan:

- Weight yourself in the morning on your bathroom smart-scale. This should take no more than 30 seconds, and the smart-scale should automatically sync the reading for the day with an online or smartphone Application.

- Track your daily diet using the Nutrition App you chose to use. This should include your beverages, breakfast, lunch, snacks and dinner. If you had saved your favorite meals on the App during the planning stage, it should take no more than a minute every day to track all your meals. If you want type in all your meals, then maybe it takes two to three minutes. No big deal. The more detailed you are when setting up the App and configuring your meal choices, the easier this daily process is.
- I recommend that you do not wait until the end of the day to track all your meals. Put in your meals as soon as you finish them. This way, before you have your next meal, you can see how many calories you have already spent and adjust accordingly. If you had a heavy breakfast and a heavy lunch, then you will have enough warning to be able to go easy on afternoon snacking and plan on a light dinner.
- Track your aerobic exercises every day. If you use a wearable device like a smartwatch, etc., then that device tracks your aerobics automatically and syncs it up with the nutrition App you are using while adjusting the total calories. Even if you track your aerobics manually on the App, it should take no more than 30 seconds to track it.
- Track your weights exercises every day. This will be as easy as checking off your exercises on the App using the exercise choices you have already saved during your planning process earlier. This tracking should take no more than 30 seconds.
- Track your sleep pattern every day using the App you have configured for that purpose. Just turn on

the App at night when you go to sleep, and stop it in the morning when you wake up.

MONTHLY ACTION ITEMS

The daily action items listed above are meant for tracking. In addition, you need to perform some monthly actions to analyze how you are doing, so that you can adjust to improve your outcomes. Here are your monthly action-items:

- Look at the monthly graph from your weight tracking App. Does it show you trending towards your ideal weight, or away from it? If you are trending in the right direction, there is no need to change anything. If not, you will need to analyze your eating and exercise patterns and optimize them.
- Your nutrition App can show you graphs of your daily calorie consumption and macro-nutrient composition. Is your calorie consumption in line with your plan? Are you consuming the planned proportions of proteins, fats and carbohydrates? Are you keeping your empty calories to a minimum? This kind of insights help you understand where you need to improve, and make those improvements consistently every month.
- Your App also shows the trending of your exercises. Are you keeping up with your exercise plans? Is life getting in the way? Having these monthly insights will help you stick to your exercise patterns more consistently.
- Analyze your sleeping patterns monthly. Are you getting enough restful sleep? Do you snore? Are you getting at least two hours of deep sleep? Is your sleep quality at 90% or above most days of the month? If not, you will need to analyze what is

wrong. Are you worrying about something that is keeping you awake at night? Do you have body aches and pains that are making sleep difficult? How comfortable are your mattress and pillows? Is your sleeping area free from other distractions? Do you have the right temperature in your bedroom? If this kind of self-analysis is not helping you improve your sleep problems, you should see a specialist.

Your monthly analysis and action items should take no more than 20 minutes every month. The idea is not to spend too much time tracking and analyzing, but rather have the Apps and devices do most of the work while you enjoy the benefits of a well-planned lifestyle with very minimal effort. Are you getting the idea?

Now, we are ready to move on to the next chapter.

MY CHECKLIST

Here is the checklist of action items for this chapter:

- I have launched my plan.
- I am tracking my daily action items
- I am tracking my monthly action-items
- I review my monthly reports and adjust my routines every month
- I find it easy to remember my daily and monthly actions and keep up with them

I am ready for the next chapter!

AUTOMATION

Automation applied to an already efficient process will magnify its benefits and makes it highly sustainable

Chapter 10
SIX STEPS TO SUSTAINABILITY

The secret to making your longevity plan sustainable is to make it automated, natural, pleasant, addictive and easy to follow.

In the previous chapters, you have spent enormous time and effort planning your approach in detail. By this time, it is quite likely that you are overwhelmed, and thinking that there are too many things to do and it is too tedious to keep up with this plan.

It does take too much determination and will power to keep up with this plan like this on an ongoing basis. What is the point of having a detailed plan if it is not sustainable, and not easy to follow?

Luckily, there is a six-step process that takes out the determination and will-power needed to follow your plan, and replaces it with unstoppable desire to keep it going. In other words, you will be addicted to your daily routines and crave them instead of having to force yourself to do them every day!

Once you read this chapter, you will realize this is the most important part of this book. The six steps are as follows:

1. Due-diligence
2. Tooling
3. Accessorizing
4. Convenience
5. Association
6. Validation

Let us consider each one of these in detail.

DUE-DILIGENCE

In the previous chapters, you spent time going through the steps for laying the foundation, being defensive and going on offensive. These three steps form a critical part of your planning process. Since planning is a one-time activity, you will need to make sure you are very detailed, honest and thorough.

In the previous chapters, I had walked you through several detailed steps for goal setting, selecting the right tools and accessories, and planning your approach in general. Please pay attention to those details and spend the time needed to complete your plan in a good way based on the advice in this book. The more detailed you are during the planning process, the easier it is going to be to implement and to keep it going. Having a detailed and practical plan is a key ingredient to making it sustainable.

TOOLING

We had discussed various tools like smart scales, nutrition, exercise and sleep management apps. Make sure you spend the time selecting and validating the right tools as described in the previous chapters. Spend the time needed to configure the tools. If you are not happy with your configuration, do it again.

If you do your due-diligence upfront, select the right tools and configure them well, managing your daily routines becomes easy, enjoyable and sustainable. You can automate most of the daily steps of your plan and keep the manual parts minimal by using the right tools.

ACCESSORIZING

We cannot always run our daily routines under ideal conditions. For example, if you walk outside as part of your aerobic exercise, the weather may often be unfriendly. Make sure you have good sneakers, suitable apparel for all kinds of weather, a good collection of music, high quality headphones, and maybe smart watches or other wearable devices. Yes, these things cost money but it is a one-time expense. What is your health and longevity worth to you?

CONVENIENCE

I cannot stress the importance of this step. As human beings, we seek convenience over perfection. Select your menu based on what is conveniently available to you. Select a health club that is convenient and close to your home or work. Set up a convenient time for your exercises. Anything this is not convenient is not sustainable and will not last.

ASSOCIATION

For your health and fitness habits to last, you should associate each habit with something that is enjoyable to you. For example, when you walk, listen to good music, walk with your dog, walk in beautiful surroundings, or walk with someone who enjoys your company. By associating your walking activity with other things you enjoy, you make it sustainable and addictive. Every health habit you have planned should be associated with things you enjoy!

If you miss your walk some days because of other priorities, you will crave to get back to it, not because you miss the walking itself but you miss listening to music or the company of your dog, or the surroundings you walk around. Associating with pleasant things makes you want to stick to your habits forever!

Some of us are very competitive. If that is you, use apps like Fitbit and Pacer that pit you against other like-minded people. These Apps allow you to compete with others so that you can motivate yourself to keep up.

VALIDATION

In one of the previous chapters, I had talked about validating your progress every month with the help of analytics, charts and graphs that your various apps, tools and devices provide you. It is necessary to check your progress every month. You should adjust and improve your results on a regular basis. If you know that you are making steady progress, accomplishing great things and feeling great while doing so, you will feel that natural motivation to keep up with your daily routines.

Better still, share your successes with your family, friends, doctor and others who care about you. The positive reinforcement form these people propels you to keep going!

This is it! This is how you make your health habits sustainable for life. I have provided you our contact information below. Please share your successes and challenges with us. You will find within us a community that is genuinely interested in helping each other, and making the best out of life. Good luck, live long, stay strong and stay healthy!

MY ACTION ITEMS

Here are the action items for this chapter:

- I have done my due-diligence with my planning and execution.
- I have selected appropriate tools to manage my goals
- I have used the right accessories to help me with my daily actions
- I have associated my daily lifestyle activities with things I love
- I validate my progress periodically and make timely adjustments as needed

This is it. You have planned and implemented the four-step plan for longevity.

Chapter 11
EXPLORING UNLIMITED POSSIBILITIES

Explore unlimited possibilities, share your successes and help your community thrive with you. Let your community lift you beyond your limitations. Give, and you shall receive!

There is one enemy of Longevity that is worse than everything else. It is loneliness. Humans are social creatures, and longevity is a team game. Every study on Longevity has pointed out the importance of family, community and a sense of belonging as major factors towards living a long and happy life.

FAMILY AND COMMUNITY

One of the previous chapters in this book talks about finding your why. There is no point in living a long life if it is not purposeful, fulfilling and fun. And this is what your family and community can give you. You can find purpose and fulfillment by being there for others, and they will undoubtedly return that favor, making your life more interesting in return.

WHY I WROTE THIS BOOK

I am fortunate to be working in a field where I get to see the impact of advances in medicine and technology on people's lives. Every day, I see more proof that people are living longer, better and happier lives because of the pioneering work being done in every area that impacts human lives.

I am also sad to see that these benefits are being enjoyed by only a select few who are fortunate to have put together a comprehensive plan for themselves. A plan that takes advantage of healthcare, technology, lifestyle changes and community living in a comprehensive and holistic manner.

I personally know a few centenarians who continue to keep tabs on latest advances in knowledge, and keep up with new things. A clear majority of people however do not have the time and tools to put together such a comprehensive plan.

This is the reason why I wrote this book. I want to share a plan that is comprehensive, but simple and easy to follow. A plan that is practical for large numbers of people regardless of their age group or the circumstances they live in. I want to keep the plan constantly updated so that people take advantage of latest advancements pertaining to longevity. Knowledge is the key!

I will fail in this effort of it is one-sided. I want to interact with you, my readers, learn about your progress and challenges, and keep making my content relevant for your needs. My goal is to genuinely help you achieve longevity, health and vibrancy in your lives.

I request you to sign up to the Facebook group I have set up for this purpose. Kindly post your progress and challenges. Interact with other members of the group. Give me feedback, and help me develop more effective products that make it attractive for people to stay on their goals and keep improving the quality of their lives. Let us make this world a better place together:

https://www.facebook.com/groups/640000990127323/.

A HUMBLE REQUEST

Thank you for reading my book!

I request you to leave me a helpful review on Amazon letting me know what you thought of the book. I appreciate your feedback and love hearing what you have to say.

I take inputs from my readers seriously, and as a result, strive to make my books better. Please know that your inputs have a direct impact towards making better content available for greater numbers of people.

Thank you so much!
I wish you good luck on your journey towards a longer, healthier and happier life!